# Dieting for Adults:

# Having That Perfect Body Shape You Wished For Is Possible

George Matthew

# Copy wright

# Table of contents

# CHAPTER 1

## Introduction To Dieting

Consuming healthy foods, beverages, and snacks, and getting regular physical activity may help you reach and maintain healthy body weight. Making suitable lifestyle choices may also help men and women prevent some health problems.

Choose whole grains more often. Try whole-wheat bread and pasta, oatmeal, or brown rice.

Select a mix of colorful vegetables. Vegetables of different colors provide a variety of nutrients. Try collards, kale, spinach, squash, sweet potatoes, and tomatoes.

At restaurants, eat only half of your meal and take the rest home.
Walk in parks, around a track, or in your neighborhood with your family or friends.
Make getting physical activity a priority.
Try to do at least 150 minutes a week of moderate-intensity aerobic activity, like biking or brisk walking.
If your time is limited, work on small amounts of activity throughout your day.
Learn more ways to move more and eat better—for yourself and your family!

## Healthy Weight

If it is tough to manage your weight, you are certainly not alone in today's world. More than 39 percent of American adults have obesity. 1 Excess weight may lead to heart disease, type 2 diabetes, kidney disease, and other chronic health problems. Setting goals to improve your health may help you lower the chances of developing weight-related health problems.

By the time you reach adulthood, 19-50years, the majority of your growth and development will be complete. This means your focus, with regards to nutritional needs, can now shift to maintaining a healthy and active lifestyle and preventing diet-related health problems, such as cardiovascular disease, hypertension and type 2 diabetes.

Consuming adequate amounts of essential vitamins, minerals, carbohydrates, fiber and protein, while limiting unhealthy fats, processed foods and added sugar, is just as important at this stage of life as it is during childhood. Overall, a healthy diet that incorporates whole grains, fruits, vegetables, lean protein and nonfat and low-fat dairy products should meet all of an adult's nutritional needs.

Dietary Recommendations for Adults

Caloric intake for adult women should be 1,800 to 2,200 calories a day and adult men should consume 2,200 to 2,800 calories depending on age and activity level. It is recommended that adults consume anywhere from 45%-65% carbohydrates, 10%-35% protein and 20%-35% of total fat, while saturated fat should be less than 10% of daily calories. You should avoid trans fats when possible, while choosing healthier fats, such as monounsaturated and polyunsaturated. Foods that include these types of fats would be nuts, seeds, fish and vegetable oils. Cholesterol intake should be less than 300 mg per day.

Here are the daily dietary recommendations for adults:

Fruits: 2 cups per day
Vegetables: 2 ½ cups per day
Dairy: 3 cups per day
Grains: 6 ounces per day
Meats and beans: 6 ounces per day
Unhealthy fats & sweets - Limit as much as possible
In addition, adult males require more of vitamins C, K, B1, B2, B3 and zinc, while women require more iron. Furthermore, pregnant women should increase their diet by 300 calories per day starting in the second trimester, while lactating women should add an additional 500 calories a day to their typical pre-pregnancy diet. Both pregnant and lactating women should make sure they consume adequate amounts of folic acid, iron and zinc.

## 3 Stages of Adulthood & Nutrition

When trying to figure out what foods to include in your diet plan, the easiest way to do it is to eat according to the nutritional recommendations for your age. After age 18, your dietary needs change as your body ages. In fact, there are three stages of adulthood that account for your body's changing nutritional needs: early adulthood, middle age and late adulthood. Each of these stages carries slightly different requirements when it comes to nutrition, although some needs may stay the same.

### Early Adulthood

According to the United States Department of Agriculture's Dietary Guidelines for 2015 to 2020, early adulthood spans from ages 19 to 30. If you fall into this age range, you should get plenty of calories to fuel your active lifestyle. In fact, it's recommended that women within this age range eat around 2,000 calories per day and that men eat between 2,600 to 3,000 calories per day for optimum health. Keep in mind that the more active you are, the more calories you should take in to stay healthy. Young adults need plenty of calories because this is traditionally when you're most active and burning the most calories each day. You'll also need to include plenty of fiber in your diet, about 28 grams per day for women and 33.6 grams for men.

## Middle Age

Middle age lasts from age 31 to 50. During this time, the body starts to slow down just a bit, so you'll want to compensate for that in your diet. The USDA recommends that women in this age range get around 1,800 calories per day and men around 2,200 to maintain their health. Eating fewer calories helps you maintain your ideal weight as your metabolism slows and you burn about 100 fewer calories per day for every decade you age. Middle age also means a little less fiber in the diet. Women should get around 25.2 grams of fiber per day and men around 30.8 grams.

Middle-aged women need higher amounts of iron in their diet to stay healthy because their bodies have low iron stores. While all adults should get 8 mg of iron per day, middle-aged women need 18 mg of iron in their diets. Lean red meats are good sources of iron, and foods rich in vitamin C aid in the absorption of the iron.

## Late Adulthood

As you enter your golden years, your body and metabolism slows down even further, so you require fewer calories to stay healthy. From age 51 on, you'll have to make some dietary adjustments. In fact, the USDA recommends that women in this age group eat around 1,600 calories per day and men eat around 2,000 per day. In terms of fiber, women need only around 22.4 grams per day and men around 28 grams per day, although eating a high-fiber diet is healthy for all adults. Older adults do need more of some nutrients like vitamin B-6 in their diets – around 1.5 mg for women and 1.7 mg for men per day.

It's important for older women to get more calcium to prevent conditions like osteoporosis as they enter menopause and experience hormonal changes. Although all adults need around 1,000 mg of calcium per day, women over 51 require 1,200 mg per day.

Adult Dietary Requirements

Many dietary requirements don't change throughout adulthood, including your protein and carbohydrate requirements. To stay healthy, all adults should aim to eat a low-sodium and low-fat diet rich in fruits and vegetables. Fruits and vegetables are rich in healthy antioxidants and wise choices at any age. During all stages of adulthood, look for foods rich in whole grains, stick to eating lean meats and don't forget to include fatty fish like salmon and sardines that are rich in omega-3 fatty acids.

# NUTRITION

## How Your Nutritional Needs Change as You Age

Eating healthy becomes especially important as you age. That's because aging is linked to a variety of changes, including nutrient deficiencies, decreased quality of life and poor health outcomes.

Luckily, there are things you can do to help prevent deficiencies and other age-related changes. For example, eating nutrient-rich foods and taking the appropriate supplements can help keep you healthy as you age.

## How Does Aging Affect Your Nutritional Needs?

Aging is linked to a variety of changes in the body, including muscle loss, thinner skin and less stomach acid.

Some of these changes can make you prone to nutrient deficiencies, while others can affect your senses and quality of life.

## Needing Fewer Calories, but More Nutrients

A person's daily calorie needs depend on their height, weight, muscle mass, activity level and several other factors.

Older adults may need fewer calories to maintain their weight, since they tend to move and exercise less and carry less muscle.

If you continue to eat the same number of calories per day as you did when you were younger, you could easily gain extra fat, especially around the belly area.

This is especially true in postmenopausal women, as the decline in estrogen levels seen during this time may promote belly fat storage.

However, even though older adults need fewer calories, they need just as high or even higher levels of some nutrients, compared to younger people.

This makes it very important for older people to eat a variety of whole foods, such as fruits, vegetables, fish and lean meats. These healthy staples can help you fight nutrient deficiencies, without expanding your waistline. Nutrients that become especially important as you age include protein, vitamin D, calcium and vitamin B12.

## You May Benefit From More Fiber

Constipation is a common health problem among the elderly. It's especially common in people over 65, and it's two to three times more common in women.

That's because people at this age tend to move less and be more likely to take medications that have constipation as a side effect. Eating fiber may help relieve constipation. It passes through the gut undigested, helping form stool and promote regular bowel movements.

# CHAPTER 2

How can you tell if you are at a healthy weight?

Your body mass index (BMI) can help you determine if you are at a healthy weight, overweight, or have obesity. BMI is a measure based on your weight about your height. You can use an online tool to calculate your BMI NIH external link. A BMI of 18.5 to 24.9 is in the healthy range. A person with a BMI of 25 to 29.9 is considered overweight. Someone with a BMI of 30 or greater is considered to have obesity.

Another important measure is your waist size. Women with a waist size of more than 35 inches, and men with a waist size of more than 40 inches, may be more likely to develop health problems. Men are more likely than women to carry extra weight around their abdomen, or belly. Extra fat, especially in the abdomen, may put people at risk for certain health problems, even if they are not overweight.

Your waist size is an important measure of whether your weight is healthy.

What are some health risks of being overweight or having obesity?

Extra weight may increase your risk for; type 2 diabetes, heart disease and stroke, high blood cholesterol, high blood pressure, kidney disease, fatty liver disease, problems with pregnancy, certain types of cancer

Why do some people become overweight?

Many factors, including consuming more calories than you need from food and beverages, lack of sleep, and low levels of physical activity, may play a part in gaining excess weight. Here are some factors that may influence weight and overall health.

The world around you. Your home, community, and workplace all may affect how you make daily lifestyle choices. Food and beverages high in fat added sugar, and calories are easy to find and sometimes hard to avoid. And they often cost less than healthier choices like fruits and vegetables. On top of that, smartphones and other devices may make it easy for you to be less active in your daily routine.

Families. Overweight and obesity tend to run in families, suggesting that genes may play a role in weight gain. Families also share food preferences and habits that may affect how much, when, and what we eat and drink.

Medicines. Some medicines, such as steroids NIH external link, and some drugs for depression NIH external link and other chronic health problems, may lead to weight gain. Ask your health care professional or pharmacist about whether weight gain is a possible side effect of medicines you are taking and if other medicines can help your health without gaining weight.

Emotions. Sometimes people snack, eat, or drink more when they feel bored, sad, angry, happy, or stressed—even when they are not hungry. Consider whether it might be your emotions making you want to eat, and try doing something else to help you cope with negative feelings or celebrate your good mood. That can help you feel better and avoid weight gain.

Lack of sleep. In general, people who get too little sleep tend to weigh more than those who get enough sleep. 2 There are several possible explanations. Sleep-deprived people may be too tired to exercise. They may take in more calories simply because they are awake longer and have more opportunities to eat. Lack of sleep may also disrupt the balance of hormones that control appetite. Researchers have noticed changes in the brains of people who are sleep deprived. These changes may spark a desire for tasty foods. 3 Learn more about sleep deprivation and deficiency NIH external link and strategies for getting enough sleep.

What kinds of foods and drinks should I consume?

Visit MyPlate.gov External link to learn more about what kinds of food and drinks to consume and what kinds to limit so you can have a healthy eating plan.

Consume more nutrient-rich foods. Nutrients—like vitamins NIH external link, minerals NIH external link, and dietary fiber—nourish our bodies by giving them what they need to be healthy. Adults are encouraged to consume some of the following foods and beverages that are rich in nutrients

fruits and vegetables
whole grains, like oatmeal, whole-grain bread, brown rice\sseafood, lean meats, poultry, and eggs
beans, peas, unsalted nuts, and seeds
sliced vegetables or baby carrots with hummus\sfat-free or low-fat milk and milk products
If you're sensitive to milk and milk products, try substituting

nondairy soy, almond, rice, or other drinks with added vitamin D and calcium\slactose-

reduced fat-free or low-fat milk
dark leafy vegetables like collard greens or kale

A display of fresh vegetables, beans, fruit, fish, lean proteins, healthy fats, whole grains, and milk.

Fruit, colorful veggies, beans, fish, and low-fat dairy products are rich sources of nutrients that give our bodies what they need to be healthy.

Consume less of these foods and beverages. Some foods and beverages have many calories but few of the essential nutrients your body needs. Added sugars and solid fats pack a lot of calories into food and beverages but provide a limited amount of healthy nutrients. Salt does not contain calories, but it tends to be in high-calorie foods. Adults should aim to limit foods and drinks such as

sugar-sweetened drinks and foods\sfoods with solid fats like butter, margarine, lard, and shortening\swhite bread, rice, and pasta that are made from refined grains\sfoods with added salt (sodium) (sodium)

whole milk
Easy snack ideas. Instead of sugary, fatty snacks, try

fat-free or low-fat milk or yogurt\sfresh or canned fruit, without added sugars
Baking dish with roasted chicken, peas, carrots, and rice.
Making better choices, like baking instead of frying chicken, can help you cut down on the added sugars and solid fats you consume.

How can I follow a healthy eating plan?
These tips may help you stay on track with your plan to eat healthier.

Reduce the overall calories you consume. If you consume more calories than you use through daily living, exercise, and other activities, it may lead to weight gain. If you consume fewer calories than you use through physical activity, it may lead to weight loss.

Have healthy snacks on hand. Whether you are at home, at work, or on the go, healthy snacks may help combat hunger and prevent overeating. Look for snacks that are low in added sugar and salt. Your best bets are whole foods—like baby carrots, fresh fruit, or low-fat or fat-free yogurt instead of chips, cakes, or cookies—rather than packaged or processed foods.

Select a mix of colorful vegetables each day. Choose dark, leafy greens—such as spinach, kale, collards, and mustard greens—and red and orange vegetables such as carrots, sweet potatoes, red peppers, and tomatoes. If you have had kidney stones, be aware that some vegetables, like spinach and sweet potatoes, are high in oxalate, a chemical that combines with calcium in urine to form a common type of kidney stone. So, if you have kidney stones, you may need to watch how much of this you eat. But for others, these are great choices. Eat a rainbow of food colors!

Choose whole grains more often. Try whole-grain bread and pasta, oatmeal, or brown rice.

A shift from solid fats to oils. Try cooking with vegetable, olive, canola, or peanut oil instead of solid fats such as butter, stick margarine, shortening, lard, or coconut oil. Choose foods that naturally contain oils, such as seafood and nuts, instead of some meat and poultry. And use salad dressings and spreads that are made with oils rather than solid fats.

Switch from frying to baking or grilling. Instead of fried chicken, try a salad topped with grilled chicken. Instead of ordering fries when eating out, ask for a side of steamed veggies.

Limit foods and beverages that are high in sugar and salt. Avoid snack foods high in salt and added sugars, and keep away from sugary soft drinks.

Read the Nutrition Facts label on packaged foods. The Nutrition Facts label tells you how many calories and servings are in a box, package, or can. The label also shows how many ingredients, such as fat, fiber, sodium, and sugar—including added sugars—are in one serving of food. You can use these facts to make healthy food choices.

Consuming food and beverages

Make a shopping list and stick to it. Don't shop when you are hungry.
Don't keep foods high in fat, added sugar, or salt in your home, workplace, or car. You can't consume what's not there! Keep healthier snacks ready so that you make the healthy choice the easy choice!
Ask for smaller servings. At a restaurant, consume only half your meal and take the rest home.
Eat your meals at a table. Turn off the TV and all other devices so you don't mindlessly eat or drink too much. Enjoy your food without distraction.
Behavior

Be realistic about weight-loss goals. Aim for a slow, modest weight loss.

Seek support. Include your family and friends.

Expect setbacks. Forgive yourself if you regain a few pounds. Adjust your plan to help you get back on track.

Add moderate- or vigorous-intensity physical activity to your weight-loss plan. This kind of activity increases your heart rate and makes you break a sweat. Examples are brisk walking, swimming, and dancing.

Sample Food and Beverage Diary

Time/ Food Feelings/ How I Can Improve

8 a.m/ Coffee with sugar and cream, oatmeal with low-fat milk, and banana Hungry. Ate my usual breakfast/ I'll keep eating breakfast every day and continue choosing whole-grain cereal and milk if I'm ever tempted by a sugary donut or high-fat breakfast sandwich.

11 a.m/ Low-fat yogurt Stomach starting to rumble/ Adding fresh fruit or whole grains will help keep me from overeating later.

12:30 p.m/ Roast beef and cheese sandwich on whole-wheat bread, potato chips, can of soda Probably ate more than I was hungry for because of the "lunch deal" the deli offered me/ If I pack my lunch, I won't be tempted in the lunch line. Choose water instead of soda.

2:30 p.m/ half chocolate bar from a coworker, large coffee with sugar and cream Feeling bored, not truly hungry. Check-in with myself to see if I am really hungry/ If I am, a snack like veggie slices with salsa or hummus is more nutritious.

7:30 p.m/ Caesar salad, dinner roll, ravioli (didn't finish the whole serving), 1/2 slice of chocolate cake Out to dinner with friends, so we all ate big portions! We split dessert, which made me feel healthy/ Next time, I'll have a salad with low-fat dressing. Good choice to split the dessert!

10:30 p.m/ Decaf herbal tea Had trouble falling asleep. Proud of myself for drinking tea rather than eating a snack/ Keep reminding yourself: Some physical activity is better than none.

Being physically active may help you start feeling better right away. It can help boost your; mood, sharpen your focus, reduce your stress, improve your sleep.

Once you are more active, keep it up with regular activities. That will improve your health even more. Studies suggest that, over time, physical activity can help you live a longer, healthier life. It may

help prevent heart disease and stroke

control your blood pressure\slower your risk of diseases like type 2 diabetes and some cancers

Man and woman powerwalking outdoors.

Getting a friend, family member, or coworker to join you may help you enjoy an activity and stick with it.

What types of physical activity do I need?

Experts recommend two types of physical activities: aerobic and muscle-strengthening activities.

Aerobic

Aerobic activities—also called endurance or cardio activities—use your large muscle groups (chest, legs, and back) to speed up your heart rate and breathing.

Aerobics can be moderate or vigorous. How can you tell what level your activity is? Take the "talk test" to find out. If you're breathing hard but can still have a conversation easily—but you can't sing—then you're doing a moderate-intensity activity. If you can only say a few words before pausing for a breath, then you're at the vigorous level. Start with moderate-intensity activities and then work up to vigorous-intensity activities to avoid injuries.

Choose aerobic activities that are fun for you. You're more likely to be active if you like what you're doing. Try getting a friend, family member, or coworker to join you. That may help you enjoy an activity and stick with it.

Try one of these activities or any others you enjoy

brisk walking or jogging\sbicycling (wear a helmet) (wear a helmet)
swimming\sdancing\splaying basketball or soccer
Regular aerobic activity can help you

manage your weight. Aerobic activity uses calories, which may help keep your weight down.

prevent heart disease and stroke NIH external link. Regular aerobic activity may strengthen your heart muscle. It may even lower your blood pressure. It may also help lower “bad” cholesterol and raise “good” cholesterol, which may lower your risk of getting heart disease.

prevent other diseases. Even moderate-intensity aerobic activity each week may lower your risk for type 2 diabetes, some cancers, anxiety, depression, Alzheimer’s disease, and other dementias

maintain strong bones. Weight-bearing aerobic activities that involve lifting or pushing your body weight, such as walking, jogging, or dancing, help to maintain strong bones.

Muscle-strengthening activity. Strength training (or resistance training) works your muscles by making you push or pull against something—a wall or floor, hand-held weights, an exercise bar, exercise bands, or even soup cans.

CHAPTER 3

## Health effects of overweight and obesity

People who have overweight or obesity*, compared to those with healthy weight, are at increased risk for many serious diseases and health conditions. These include:

High blood pressure (hypertension) (hypertension).
High LDL cholesterol, low HDL cholesterol, or high levels of triglycerides (dyslipidemia) (dyslipidemia).
Type 2 diabetes.
Coronary heart disease.
Stroke.
Gallbladder disease.

Osteoarthritis (a breakdown of cartilage and bone within a joint) (a breakdown of cartilage and bone within a joint).
Sleep apnea and breathing problems.
Many types of cancer.
Low quality of life.
Mental illnesses such as clinical depression, anxiety, and other mental disorders.
Body pain and difficulty with physical functioning

Overweight is defined as a body mass index (BMI) of 25 or higher. Obesity is defined as a BMI of 30 or higher. See the BMI calculator for people 20 years and older and the BMI calculator for people ages 2 through 19.
The latest WHO projections indicate that at least one in three of the world's adult population is overweight and almost one in 10 is obese. Additionally, there are over 40 million children under age five who are overweight.

Being overweight or obese can have a serious impact on health. Carrying extra fat leads to serious health consequences such as cardiovascular disease (mainly heart disease and stroke), type 2 diabetes, musculoskeletal disorders like osteoarthritis, and some cancers (endometrial, breast, and colon) (endometrial, breast, and colon). These conditions cause premature death and substantial disability.

What is not widely known is that the risk of health problems starts when someone is only very slightly overweight and that the likelihood of problems increases as someone becomes more and more overweight. Many of these conditions cause long-term suffering for individuals and families. In addition, the costs for the health care system can be extremely high.

The good news is that being overweight and obese are largely preventable. The key to success is to achieve an energy balance between calories consumed on one hand, and calories used on the other hand.

To reach this goal, people can limit energy intake from total fats and shift fat consumption away from saturated fats to unsaturated fats; increase consumption of fruit and vegetables, as well as legumes, whole grains, and nuts; and limit their intake of sugars. And to increase calories used, people can boost their levels of physical activity - to at least 30 minutes of regular, moderate-intensity activity on most days.

CHAPTER 4

## Dieting Tips For Adults; 22 Ways to Stay on Track

Tip No. 1: Drink plenty of water or other calorie-free beverages.

Before you tear into that bag of potato chips, drink a glass of water first. People sometimes confuse thirst with hunger, so you can end up eating extra calories when an ice-cold glass of water is all you needed. If plain water doesn't cut it, try drinking flavored sparkling water or brewing a cup of fruit-infused herbal tea.

Tip No. 2: Be choosy about nighttime snacks.

Mindless eating occurs most frequently after dinner when you finally sit down and relax. Snacking in front of the TV is one of the easiest ways to throw your diet off course. Either close down the kitchen after a certain hour or allow yourself a low-calorie snack, like a 100-calorie pack of cookies or a half-cup scoop of low-fat ice cream.

Tip No. 3: Enjoy your favorite foods.

Instead of cutting out your favorite foods altogether, be a slim shopper. Buy one fresh bakery cookie instead of a box, or a small portion of candy from the bulk bins instead of a whole bag. You can still enjoy your favorite foods – the key is moderation.

Tip No. 4: Eat several mini-meals during the day.

If you eat fewer calories than you burn, you'll lose weight. But when you're hungry all the time, eating fewer calories can be a challenge. "Studies show people who eat 4-5 meals or snacks per day are better able to control their appetite and weight," says obesity researcher Rebecca Reeves, DrPH, RD. She recommends dividing your daily calories into smaller meals or snacks and enjoying most of them earlier in the day – dinner should be the last time you eat.

Tip No. 5: Eat protein at every meal.

Protein is the ultimate fill-me-up food – it's more satisfying than carbs or fats and keeps you feeling full for longer. It also helps preserve muscle mass and encourages fat burning. So be sure to incorporate healthy proteins like seafood, lean meat, egg whites, yogurt, cheese, soy, nuts, or beans into your meals and snacks.

Tip No. 6: Spice it up.

Add spices or chilies to your food for a flavor boost that can help you feel satisfied. "Food that is loaded with flavor will stimulate your taste buds and be more satisfying, so you won't eat as much," says American Dietetic Association spokeswoman Malena Perdomo, RD. When you need something sweet, suck on a red-hot fireball candy. It's sweet, spicy, and low in calories.

Tip No. 7: Stock your kitchen with healthy, convenient foods.

Having ready-to-eat snacks and meals-in-minutes on hand sets you up for success. You'll be less likely to hit the drive-through or order a pizza if you can throw together a healthy meal in five or 10 minutes. Here are some essentials to keep on hand: frozen vegetables, whole-grain pasta, reduced-fat cheese, canned tomatoes, canned beans, pre-cooked grilled chicken breast, whole grain tortillas or pitas, and bags of salad greens.

Tip No. 8: Order children's portions at restaurants.

Ordering a child-size entree is a great way to cut calories and keep your portions reasonable. This has become such a popular trend that most servers won't bat an eye when you order off the kids' menu. Another trick is to use smaller plates. This helps the portions look like more, and if your mind is satisfied, your stomach likely will be, too.

Tip No. 9: Swap a cup of pasta for a cup of vegetables.

Simply by eating less pasta or bread and more veggies, you could lose a dress or pants size in a year. "You can save from

100-200 calories if you reduce the portion of starch on your plate and increase the number of vegetables," says Cynthia Sass, RD, a spokeswoman for the Academy of Nutrition and Dietetics.

Tip No. 10: Always eat breakfast.

It seems like an easy diet win: Skip breakfast and you'll lose weight. Yet many studies show the opposite can be true. Not eating breakfast can make you hungry later, leading to too much nibbling and binge eating at lunch and dinner. To lose weight — and keep it off — always make time for a healthy morning meal, like high-fiber cereal, low-fat milk, and fruit.

Tip No. 11: Include fiber in your diet.

Fiber Aids digestion prevents constipation, lowers cholesterol — and can help with weight loss. Most Americans get only half the fiber they need. To reap fiber's benefits, most women should get about 25 grams daily, while men need about 38 grams – or 14 grams per 1,000 calories. Good fiber sources include oatmeal, beans, whole grain foods, nuts, and most fruits and vegetables.

Tip No. 12 Clean the cupboard of fattening foods

If you have chips in the pantry and ice cream in the freezer, you're making weight loss harder than it has to be. Reduce temptation by purging the cupboards of fattening foods. Want an occasional treat? Make sure you have to leave the house to get it – preferably by walking.

Tip No. 13: Lose weight slowly.

If you're losing weight but not as fast as you'd like, don't get discouraged. Dropping pounds takes time, just like gaining them did. Experts suggest setting a realistic weight loss goal of about one to two pounds a week. If you set your expectations too high, you may give up when you don't lose weight fast enough. Remember, you start seeing health benefits when you've lost just 5 percent -10 percent of your body weight.

Tip No. 14: Weigh yourself once a week.

People who weigh themselves regularly tend to have more weight loss success. But most experts suggest weighing yourself only once a week, so you're not derailed by daily fluctuations. When you weigh yourself, follow these tips: Weigh yourself at the same time of day, on the same day of the week, on the same scale, and in the same clothes.

Tip No. 15: Get enough sleep.

When you're sleep deprived, your body overproduces the appetite-stimulating hormone ghrelin but underproduces the hormone leptin, which tells you when you're full. Getting enough sleep may make you feel rested and full and keep you from doing unnecessary snacking.

Tip No. 16: Understand portion sizes.

We're so used to super-sizing when we eat out that it's easy to carry that mindset home. To right-size, your diet, use a kitchen scale and measuring cups to measure your meals for a week or two. Use smaller plates and glasses to downsize your portions. Split restaurant servings in half — making two meals out of one big one. Portion out snack servings instead of eating them directly from the container.

Tip No. 17: Eat more fruits and vegetables.

The best "diet" is one where you get to eat more food, not less. If you eat more fruits and vegetables, you shouldn't feel as hungry because these nutrient-rich foods are also high in fiber and water, which can give you a feeling of fullness. Snacking can be a good thing as long as you choose smart snacks.

Tip No. 18: Limit alcohol to weekends.

Alcohol contains empty calories: a five-ounce glass of wine has 125, and a bottle of beer about 153. Because our bodies don't require those calories, they can get converted into fat. If you enjoy an occasional drink, consider a compromise. Enjoy your favorite alcoholic beverage on weekends only, with just one drink for women per day, and two for men.

Tip No. 19: Chew sugarless gum.
The next time you want to grab a fattening snack, reach for some sugar-free gum instead. Chewing some types of gum gives

you fresh breath and can also help manage hunger, control snack cravings, and aid in weight loss. (Keep in mind, however, that excess sorbitol, a sugar alcohol sometimes used in low-calorie gums, can have a laxative effect in some people.) Although gum might make you eat less, it doesn't mean you can stop eating right. A good diet and exercise are still important.

Tip No. 20: Keep a food diary.

A simple pen and paper can dramatically boost your weight loss. Studies show the act of writing down what you eat and drink tends to make you more aware of what, when, and how much you're consuming – leading you to ultimately take in fewer calories. One study found that people who kept a food diary six days a week lost about twice as much as those who only kept a diary one day a week or less.

Tip No. 21: Celebrate success (but not with food)

You lost five pounds this month and walked every other day? Time to celebrate! Rewarding weight loss success really can encourage more success, so revel in your achievements. Buy a CD, take in a movie, and set a prize for the next milestone. Just don't celebrate with a sundae or deep-dish pizza.

Tip No. 22: Get help from family and friends.

Getting support can help you reach your weight loss goals. So tell family and friends about your efforts to lead a healthy lifestyle. Maybe they'll join you in exercising, eating right, and losing weight. When you feel like giving up, they'll help you, keep you honest, and cheer you on – making the whole experience a lot easier.

www.ingramcontent.com/pod-product-compliance
Lightning Source LLC
LaVergne TN
LVHW020524160826
845677LV00015B/3881

* 9 7 9 8 8 4 4 2 5 3 0 5 8 *